Moving Right Along After Open Heart Surgery

a book for patient and family education

by

Susan G. Burrows, R.N., M.N.

and

Carole A. Gassert, R.N., Ph.D.

We express appreciation to those professionals and patients who helped us review this material.

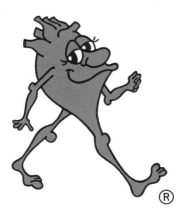

More about the authors:

Susan Burrows, R.N., M.N., is a Clinical Nurse Specialist in Cardiovascular Surgery at Emory University Hospital in Atlanta, GA. Besides this book, she is coauthor with Carole Gassert of *Going For Heart Surgery* and has developed numerous booklets, including one on heart transplantation, and audiovisual programs for patient education. The Open Heart Surgery Education Program at Emory, of which she is a part, has received national recognition by the American Hospital Association. She has also served as a speaker at many cardiovascular conferences.

Carole Gassert, R.N., Ph.D., is an Assistant Professor of Nursing Informatics at the University of Maryland School of Nursing. For many years, she served as Clinical Nurse Specialist at the University of Virginia Hospital and Crawford W. Long Memorial Hospital of Emory University. Also, she has taught cardiac nursing at the University of Virginia and Georgia State University. Besides this book and the patient book, *Going For Heart Surgery*, Carole has contributed to the *American Journal of Nursing, Computers in Nursing* and to the nursing book, *Practices.*

Published and distributed by:
Pritchett & Hull Associates, Inc.

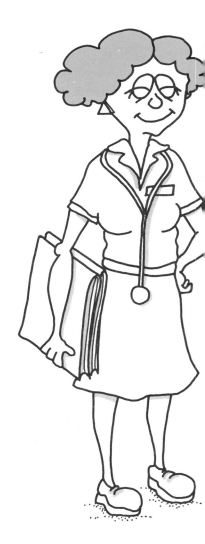

Introduction

Your recovery is on its way, and, as you think about going home, you may have many questions. *"When can I drive?" "Will I be on a special diet?" "When can I have sex?"* This book answers these questions and many more. It also reviews what you have learned about your heart and open heart surgery.

Talking about your surgery with others is OK if you remember that each person's recovery is different. No one has the same medicines, activities and recovery rate. How fast you recover depends on the type of heart surgery you had and how active you were before your surgery. You will get stronger, and your confidence and well-being will return.

We wish you a smooth recovery.

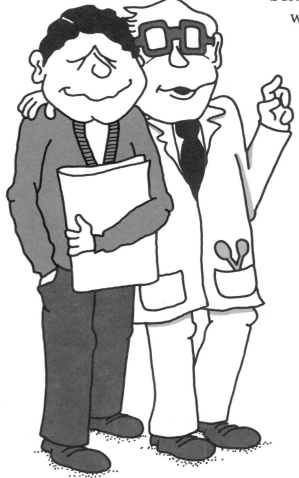

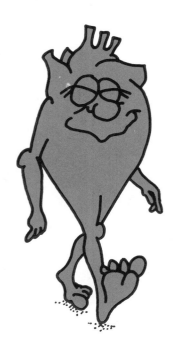

Contents

Going home

On the day of discharge, plan your activities so that you can get a lot of rest. The excitement of going home can be very tiring. When you get home, you may need a nap.

Getting ready to go home may increase the soreness in your chest. You may want to ask your nurse for pain medicine just before leaving the hospital.

Car: There is no need to go home in an ambulance. Riding in a car is best because you can stop often to stretch your legs or rest. A pillow and blanket and loose fitting clothes may make your trip more comfortable. Be sure to use your **seat belt** and **shoulder strap** in the car.

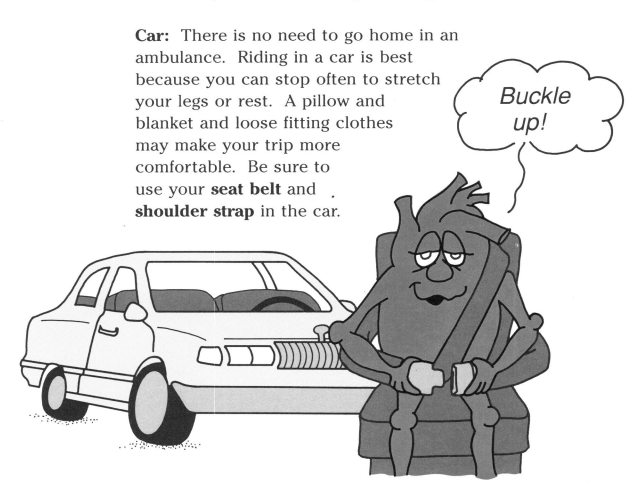

Buckle up!

Airplane: If you fly home, plan for help with your bags and transportation at the airport. If the flight is long, change positions and do your leg exercises to help the blood flow in your legs.

Getting back to normal

At times, your recovery may seem to be slow. You may feel drained from limited activity, lack of good sleep, medicines and surgery itself. On some days you will have more energy than on others. This is all normal.

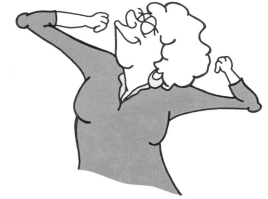

Your emotions

It's normal after surgery to have a "let down" or depressed feeling. It takes a lot of energy to deal with fear and anxiety, and you may show your feelings more than usual. You may be tearful or cry. At times you may be irritable. Some people have bad dreams. Others have a loss of memory or can't concentrate. You may be embarrassed or worry about your feelings. These emotions should go away by the end of your recovery (4 to 6 weeks). If they don't, call your doctor.

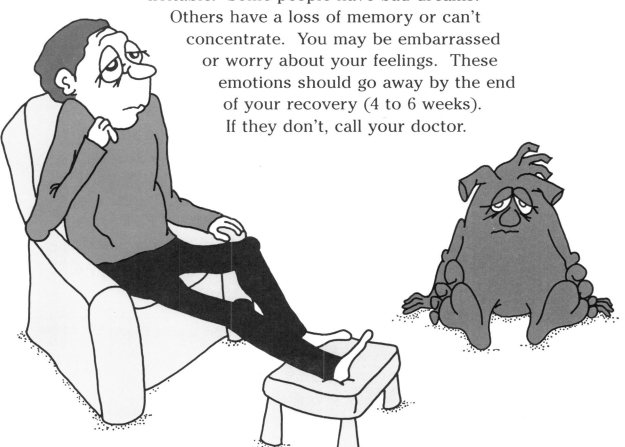

Your body

Recovery from heart surgery is 4 to 6 weeks. During this time, you start to build up your strength and get back to your normal day.

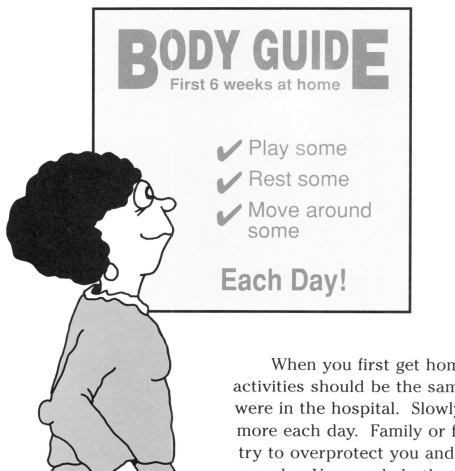

BODY GUIDE
First 6 weeks at home

✔ Play some
✔ Rest some
✔ Move around some

Each Day!

When you first get home your activities should be the same as they were in the hospital. Slowly do a little more each day. Family or friends may try to overprotect you and limit what you do. You can help them by sharing this book and letting them know how much activity is OK.

Use common sense. Set goals that you can reach. You don't want to overdo it, but you don't want to be inactive either. Rest when you are tired. Change an activity when it makes you tired. Doing too much at this time will not hurt your heart, but it will cause fatigue.

Incisions

During the first weeks after surgery, your incision may be bruised. It may also itch, feel numb or be sore. In just a few weeks the scar will begin to look better. Changes in the weather, too much (or too little) activity and sleeping in one position can cause soreness. At times your back or shoulders may also feel sore, and you may notice a swelling or lump at the top of your chest incision. All of these things are common and will slowly go away.

For back and shoulder soreness, some people use a heating pad on LOW. Maintain good posture, and move your neck and shoulder muscles in a normal way. This will help you to be less stiff. A mild pain reliever may also help with discomfort.

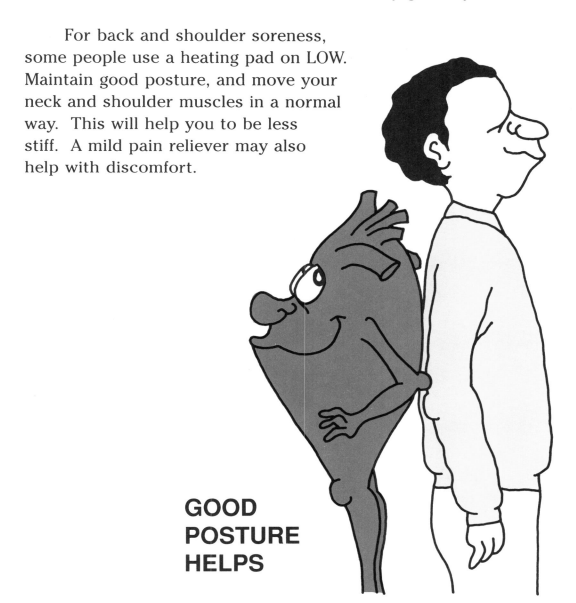

GOOD POSTURE HELPS

Sternum (breastbone)

Your main cautions after surgery relate to healing of the sternum. This bone is held together by wires, but you can't feel them. These wires don't have to be removed, but they will show up on X rays.

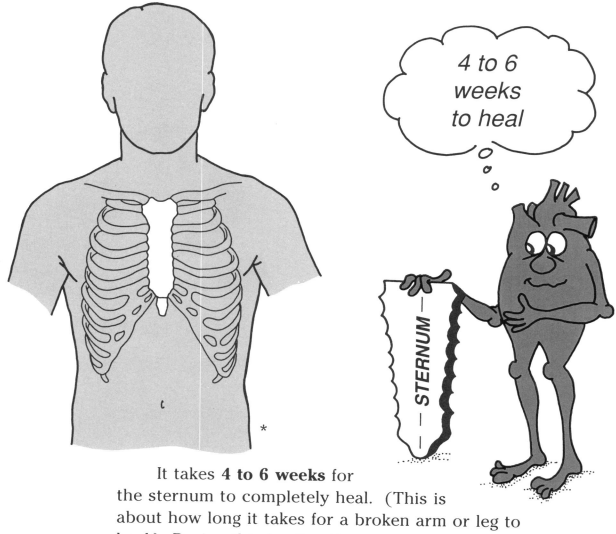

It takes **4 to 6 weeks** for the sternum to completely heal. (This is about how long it takes for a broken arm or leg to heal.) During this healing time you may notice a slight clicking or movement of the sternum when you breathe or turn. This is common and should go away when your sternum heals.

* Illustration from *Medical Art, graphics for use,* Williams & Wilkens Co., Baltimore, © 1982. Used with permission.

Bathing

You can bathe **when the incision is healed.** At first you may be weak so have someone close by to help you if needed. Until you feel stronger, it may help to place a chair in the shower. Use a heavy chair or one with rubber tips on the legs. You don't want the chair to move around while in the shower.

Do not bathe in very hot water. It may cause you to feel dizzy or weak.

Wash your incision gently with soap, but do not scrub. If strips of tape have been placed on your incision, remove them 4 to 5 days after you go home.

Use a soap that does <u>not</u> contain skin softener
(i.e. Dove)

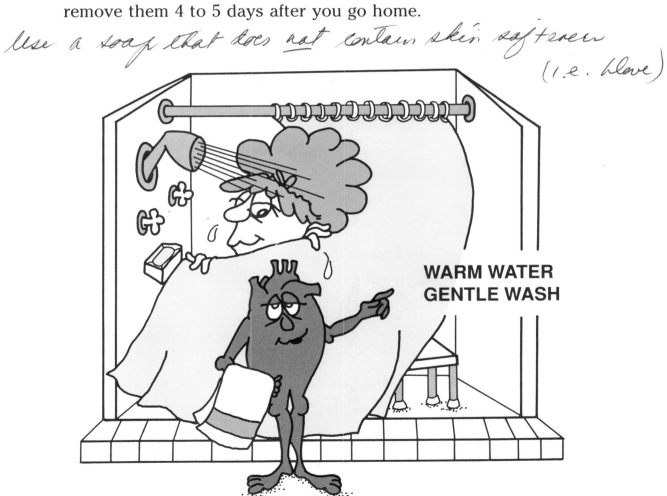

WARM WATER GENTLE WASH

Diet

Eating well-balanced meals will speed your healing and make you less tired after surgery. Your appetite may be down, but it will pick up as you start to recover. If you have been put on a special diet, ask your nurse or dietitian to explain anything that you don't understand.

A healthy heart diet is one that is low in cholesterol, saturated fat, sugar, sodium and caffeine. You will not have to eat a lot of new or strange foods if you don't want to. You may only have to make a few changes. Most people find out that they can keep eating what they like once they learn how to fix foods in more healthy ways.

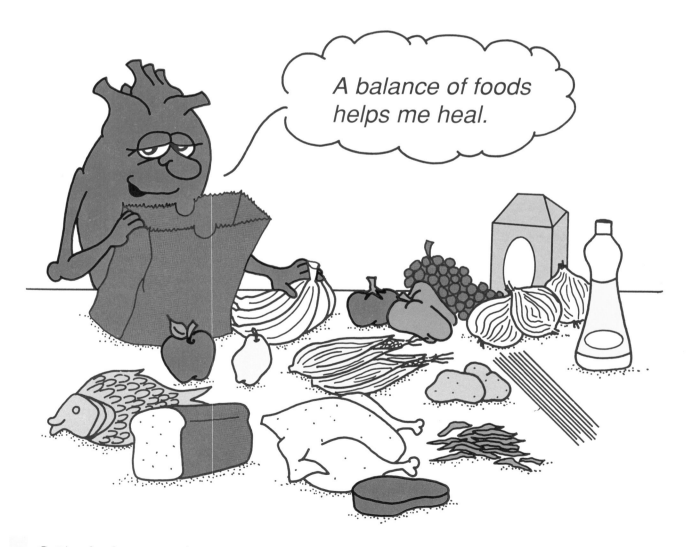

A balance of foods helps me heal.

One way to learn about foods is to **buy a heart cookbook.** These cookbooks give you the fat, cholesterol, sodium, protein, carbohydrate and caloric content of foods. They also tell you how to season foods, make sauces and eat out with less fat and cholesterol. (See p. 56.)

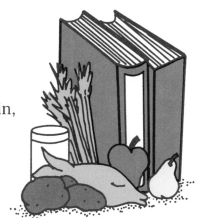

Reading labels is another way to learn about foods. Don't buy foods that list: palm oil, coconut oil or hydrogenated oil. These are bad for you (saturated fats). **Don't be fooled.** The front of a food label may say: "natural," "no cholesterol" or "healthy snack." But when you turn it over, the back label lists one of the saturated oils. It's the **combination of saturated fat and cholesterol** that clogs the arteries.

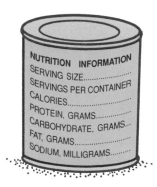

Cooking

Use **small amounts** of vegetable oil in salads or in cooking. Safflower, corn, soy, sunflower, peanut, canola and olive oils are OK. So is a non-stick spray.

Bake, broil, steam, poach or grill. Don't fry. Cook with very little salt (or none), and don't add more salt at the table. Season with herbs, fruits, vegetables and no-salt products.

Eat very few egg yolks—4 or less a week (including the eggs used in fixing other foods). Egg whites are OK. So are egg substitutes. You can cook with these or eat them in place of egg yolks.

More about *cholesterol*

Cholesterol is found in **animal foods**. The body uses it to make some hormones and help us burn food. Cholesterol is carried in the blood by lipoproteins. HDL's (high density lipoproteins) are thought to remove cholesterol from the blood before it builds up in the arteries. LDL's (low density lipoproteins) add to fatty buildup in the arteries. Your aim is to have a total blood cholesterol of less than 200 with HDL's of 50 to 70. Your doctor can tell you more about these numbers.

More about *saturated fats*

Saturated fats are found in **animal and plant foods.** These fats are **solid at room temperature.** Foods like butter, hard margerines, Crisco and the solid layer of grease that forms when a stew or broth cools are saturated fats. Cream, half and half, whole milk, ice cream, sour cream and most cheeses also have a lot of saturated fat.

A dietitian can tell you how many grams of fat to eat a day.

Alcohol

Drink only if you have no addiction problem. Drink no more than: 2 oz of 80 proof whiskey or 7 oz of wine or 17 oz of beer in any one day. Too much alcohol is known to weaken the heart muscle.

If you are on tranquilizers, sleeping pills or pain medicine of any kind, don't drink. Alcohol increases the side effects of these drugs.

Driving

Do not drive a car for about 4 to 6 weeks after surgery. During recovery your reaction time will be slowed due to weakness, fatigue or medication. And it takes time for your sternum (breastbone) to heal. Even if you were wearing a seat belt to drive and had an accident, you could hit the steering wheel and reinjure your sternum. Reinjury could also be caused by riding: bikes, motorcycles, horses, lawn mowers, snowmobiles or tractors.

You can ride in a car, but long trips should be put off until after the return visit to your surgeon. When riding, **stop every 1 to 2 hours and walk around.** This will improve blood flow in your legs and help prevent swelling.

She breaks for boogie!

Exercise

Exercise improves muscle tone and strength after surgery. It also helps you feel better about yourself. Before you begin to exercise, think about these:

- It takes time to get your strength back after surgery. Be patient.
- Exercise when you are rested.
- Warm up before you exercise.

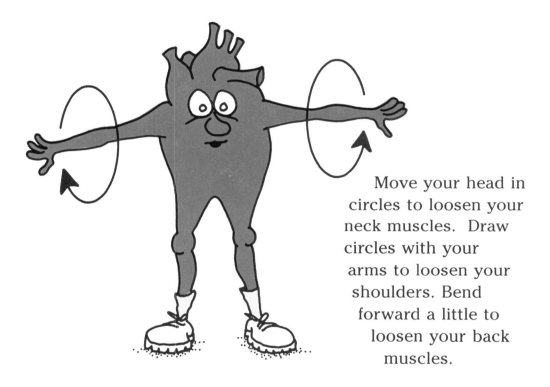

Move your head in circles to loosen your neck muscles. Draw circles with your arms to loosen your shoulders. Bend forward a little to loosen your back muscles.

- Cool down after exercise by walking slowly for 3 to 5 minutes.
- Stop exercising at the first sign of angina, severe fatigue or shortness of breath.

Some people join a cardiac rehab program. These programs teach you how to exercise safely and help you learn how to have a more healthy lifestyle.

Do the amount and kind of exercise your doctor suggests. He or she may have you start a walking program or ride a stationary bike.

Walking

Start walking at home on a flat surface. It takes less energy to walk on level ground than to walk up a hill. If you must walk up and down hills, shorten the distance. You may want to get someone to drive you to a shopping mall, recreation center or track to walk.

You will get less tired and enjoy a walk more if you wear **comfortable shoes.** Use non-skid soles to help prevent falls.

Exercise can be done almost anywhere, but these make it harder:

- very hot or cold weather
- very humid weather
- strong winds
- high altitude
- air pollution

Slowly add to your distance over the next month. Increase your speed slowly. **How far and how fast you walk** is what helps the heart get stronger.

Ask your doctor for a walking program that fits what you can do.

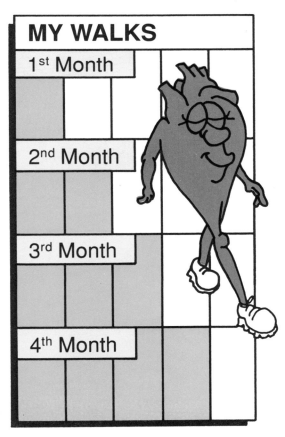

MY WALKS

1st Month

2nd Month

3rd Month

4th Month

Build up slowly.

See page 52.

Stationary bike

Many people like to work out on a stationary bike. You don't have to worry about hills or bad weather, and you can listen to music or watch TV while you ride.

Set a comfortable temperature in your exercise room. Move the seat of the bike to a good height for you. Your knees should be slightly bent when you pedal.

While riding:

- relax your body
  - lean forward slightly
    - keep a slight bend in your knee
      - pedal on the ball of your foot

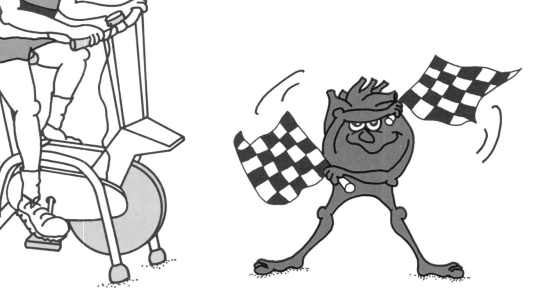

The distance and speed that you pedal decide how strong your heart gets from this workout. Pedal, rest, then pedal again. Ask your doctor for a bike program that is right for you.

See page 53.

When to stop exercise

Your body may tell you to stop exercising by giving you the following warning signs:

Heart	**Lungs**	**Muscles**
• chest pain	• trouble breathing	• muscle strain
• irregular heartbeats	• shortness of breath	• pulling on breastbone
• dizziness		

If you get any of these signs, stop working out. If they do not go away with rest, call your doctor.

If you have chest pain or an irregular heartbeat, let your doctor know (even if it does go away with rest).

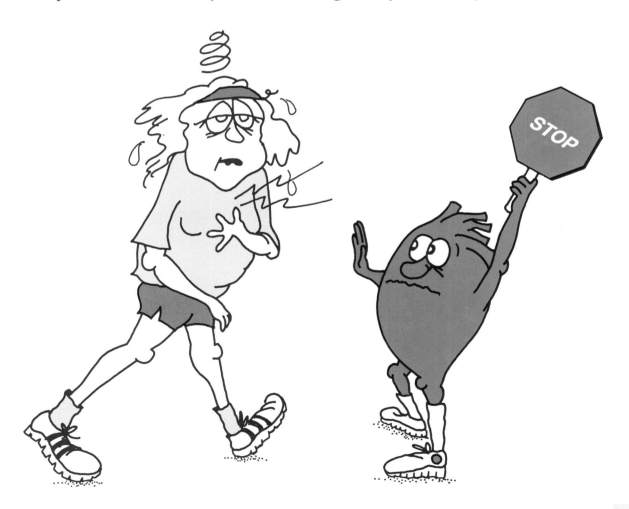

Household chores

Wait until after your 4 to 6 weeks checkup or when your doctor says it is OK to begin household duties (child care, making meals, etc).

During the first 2 weeks at home, as you get stronger, you may feel like:

- setting and clearing the table
- minor repairs around the house
- dusting furniture
- potting plants
- shopping

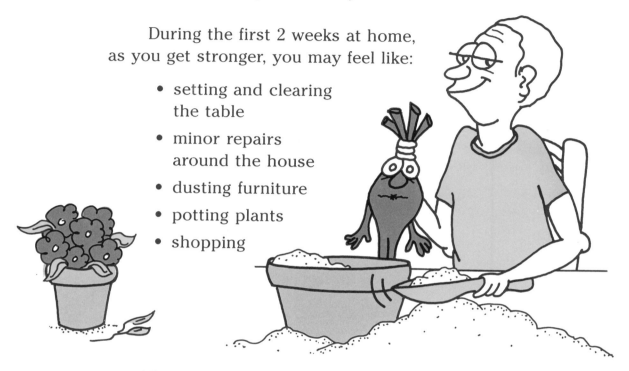

The actions listed below put stress on the breastbone and take more energy. **Don't** do these until you have healed or until your doctor says it is OK:

- vacuuming
- moving furniture
- weeding
- raking or mowing the lawn
- gardening
- mopping
- lifting and carrying items that weigh more than 5 to 10 lbs

Anything that is very tiring or causes discomfort should be stopped until after recovery.

Lifting

Do not lift more than 5 to 10 lbs for 4 to 6 weeks after surgery. Lifting strains your breastbone. Do not lift such things as:

- suitcases
- groceries
- children
- pets
- large purses or briefcases

Also, there are other things that can put strain on your breastbone.

Don't try to:

- open stuck windows
- unscrew jar lids
- push or pull open heavy doors
- move heavy furniture

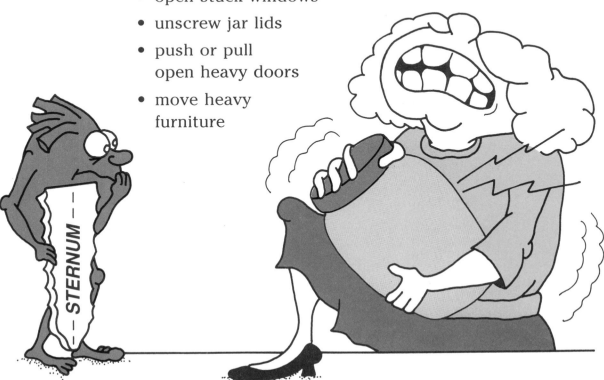

Medications

You may need medication after open heart surgery. Many people do. Your doctor may even prescribe the same drugs after surgery that you were taking before. You may also receive medicines for pain.

Know these about any medicine you take:

- the name
  - what it does
    - how much to take
      - when and how to take it
        - side effects

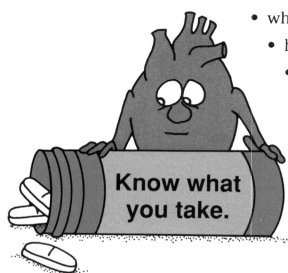

Know what you take.

Do not increase, decrease or stop your medicine without your doctor's OK. If you should forget and miss a pill, don't take 2 the next time.

Your medicines are prescribed just for you and may be harmful to someone else. **Do not let anyone else take your medicine.**

Drugs can cause side effects. Call your doctor right away if you develop any of these:

- rash
- wheezing
- fever
- dizziness
- severe bruising

- nausea/vomiting
- diarrhea
- irregular heartbeats
- severe headache
- jaundice
  ("yellow" skin, eyes, etc.)

Keep all medicines away from children.

Take only the medicine prescribed at the time you leave the hospital. Medicine taken before your surgery should not be continued unless your doctor says it's OK.

Have your prescriptions filled at your local drugstore so that it will be easy to have them refilled as needed. If you need to have any of these explained again, ask your druggist when you have the prescriptions filled.

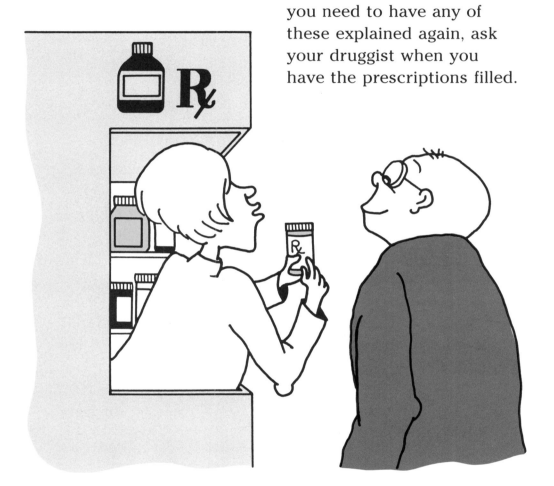

As drugs become outdated they may be useless or even harmful. The expiration date most often is on the bottle. If your drug is more than a few months old, ask your druggist if it is still good.

Keep your medicine in the container it came in. Be sure the name and dose is on the label.

Recreation

Once you are home and feeling stronger, you may enjoy dining out, going to a movie, getting your hair styled or making short shopping trips. But keep in mind that you have been less active for some time. Pay attention to how you feel. You will be the best judge of when it is time to rest or do the activities your doctor suggests.

When you first get home, you may enjoy:

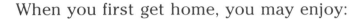

- an easy walk
- cards
- theaters or movies
- fishing (from a bank or bridge)
- golf (putting practice)
- wading (lake, pool or calm ocean)
- needlework
- painting pictures
- croquet
- photography
- spectator sports (when you won't get tired in large crowds)

After your recovery is complete, your doctor may say that you can:

- play a full game of golf
- play tennis
- fish from a boat
- hunt
- swim
- horseback ride
- take a brisk walk
- jog

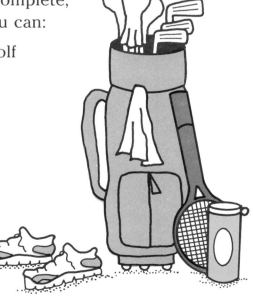

Rest

Right now, your body treats all activity as "work." Routines like bathing, shaving or brushing your hair can be tiring. You need rest to help get your strength back.

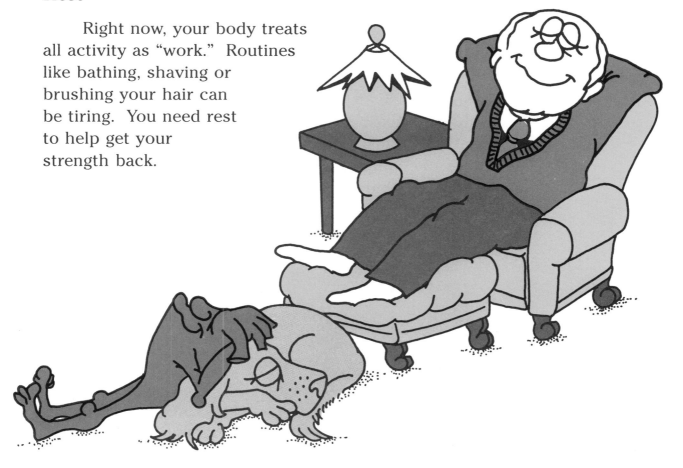

To get the rest needed:

- Plan two 20 to 30 minute rest times each day during the first week or two at home. **You don't need to go to bed, just rest.**

- Rest between play or work to keep from getting too tired.

- Try to get 8 to 10 hours of sleep each night. Don't stay up late one night and try to "catch up" the next. If you must stay up late, take a nap earlier in the evening.

- Look at your progress **one day at a time.** Don't push yourself or compare yourself to others. It takes time to regain your strength.

Sex

Just about everyone worries about having sex after open heart surgery. This includes both the person who had the surgery and his or her partner. Will sex injure the breastbone? Will sex damage the heart? Will I be able to perform? These are normal things to consider but not to worry about. It takes about the same energy to have sex as it does to climb 2 flights of stairs. So if you feel good and are rested, then sex can be enjoyed as much after surgery as it was before. Here are some things to keep in mind:

- If you are tired and tense, wait until you feel better.

- If you use positions that pull on your chest and cause discomfort, try others.

- If you feel uneasy before sex, allow more time for hugging and caressing. **Relax and get in touch with your partner again.**

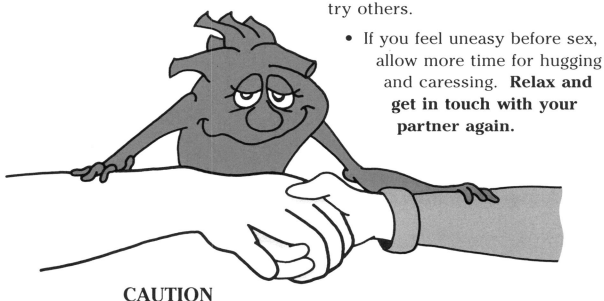

CAUTION

A woman should not plan to have a baby until recovery from surgery is complete. Most doctors advise waiting at least 1 year. In some cases, a woman should not get pregnant after heart surgery. Certain contraceptives cannot be used by heart patients. Ask about birth control or pregnancy before you leave the hospital.

Smoking

For some of you, surgery forced you to stop smoking. It is very important that you keep on NOT SMOKING. Studies show that smoking can increase heart rate, narrow blood vessels, raise blood pressure, cause spasms of the coronary arteries and scar the lungs. It may be hard not to smoke again, but you CAN do it. Smoking is the worst thing you can do to your heart.

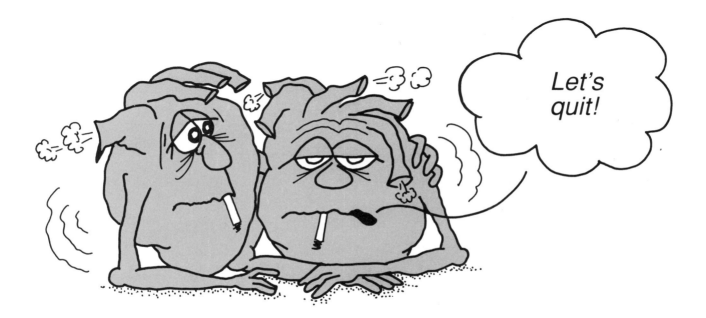

Here are some tips to help you not smoke:

- Ask family and friends not to smoke around you.

- Each day say, "I won't smoke today." Don't set yourself up to fail by saying, "I'll never smoke again." And don't think, "One little smoke won't matter." It will.

- Do things with your hands, like puzzles or needlepoint.

continued next page

- Change the habits that make you want to smoke. For example, don't linger at the table after a meal.

- Avoid high calorie snacks. Nibble on foods like carrots, celery sticks and fruits.

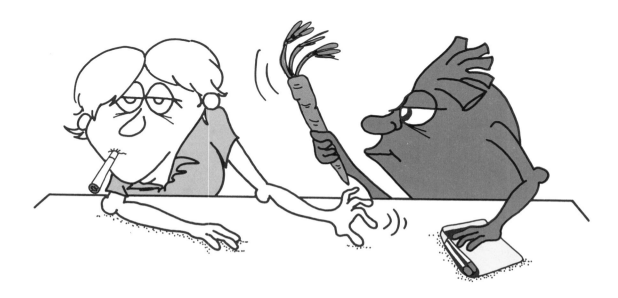

- Keep a clean mouth taste. Brush your teeth after eating, and use a mouthwash.

- Avoid coffee, alcohol or other drinks that make you want to smoke.

- When you are tempted to smoke, chew sugarless gum or play with a paper clip or marble. If your hands and mouth are busy, you will be less likely to light up.

- If you can't quit alone, call your hospital, clinic, heart or lung association. Ask if there is a stop-·smoking program or other support group to help you quit.

Often it takes more than one effort to stop smoking. Keep trying until you win the battle.

Stairs

You can climb stairs, but take your time and go slowly. Climbing stairs takes more energy than walking. At first it may be less tiring if you plan your day so that you go up and down stairs less often. If you have an upstairs bedroom, there is no need to change where you sleep.

Sit down and rest if you become

- tired
- short of breath or
- dizzy

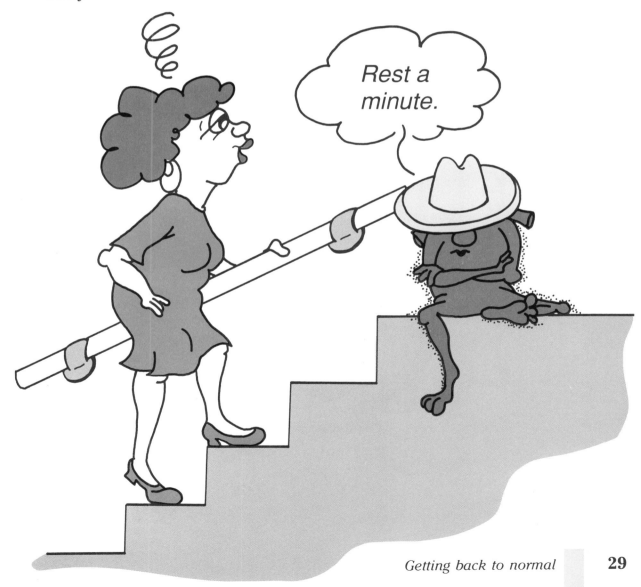

Support stockings

You may be asked to wear support stockings during the first part of your recovery when you are less active. These stockings **aid blood flow** and help **reduce swelling** in the legs.

- Keep wearing the stockings your first few weeks at home or until your activity is back to normal.

- To avoid strain or discomfort to your incision, ask a family member to put them on you.

- Be sure to get all wrinkles out of the stockings so there won't be any pressure areas.

- Don't cross your legs when sitting. Crossed legs put pressure on the areas behind your knees and decrease blood flow in your legs.

If you have a problem with swelling of your legs:

- keep on wearing the stockings

- raise your legs when sitting

- don't stand for long periods of time

Visitors

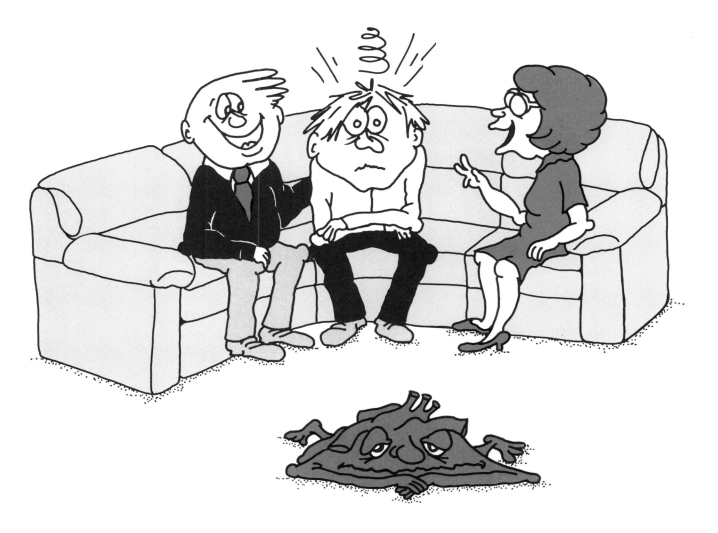

Visitors mean well. They care about you and want to see how you are doing. But too much "visiting" can be very tiring and get in the way of your recovery. So can too many phone calls.

During your first 2 weeks at home, discourage a lot of visits from relatives and friends. **About 2 short visits a day is enough.** Let them know that rest is an important part of your recovery. And don't be afraid to excuse yourself from company when you feel tired and need to rest.

When to visit your doctor

A report of your surgery and progress will be sent to your local doctor. Call him or her when you get home. Your own doctor will most likely make an appointment to see you within 2 weeks.

S	M	T	W	TH	F	S
			SEE DOC			
		SEE SURGEON				

Set a time to see your surgeon or cardiologist in about 4 weeks.

When to call your doctor

If any symptoms concern you, call your local doctor. If you can't reach him or her, call your surgeon or cardiologist.

Call if you have any of these:

- redness, swelling, extreme tenderness or drainage from incision

  (Some clear drainage from the leg incision is common, but report **ANY** drainage from the chest.)

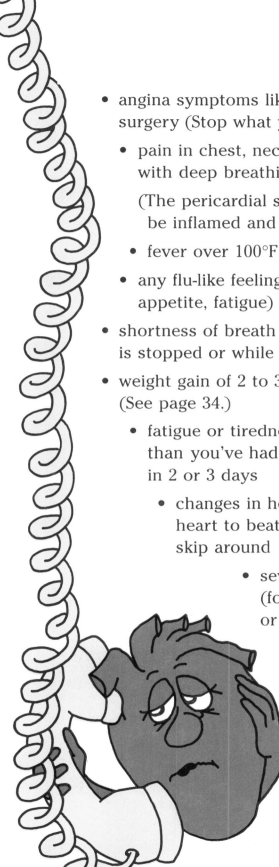

- angina symptoms like those you had before surgery (Stop what you are doing and take NTG.)

  - pain in chest, neck or shoulder that is worse with deep breathing

    (The pericardial sac which covers the heart can be inflamed and irritated after surgery.)

  - fever over 100°F for more than 2 or 3 days

  - any flu-like feelings (aches, chills, fever, loss of appetite, fatigue) that last 2 or 3 days

- shortness of breath that goes on after an activity is stopped or while you are at rest

- weight gain of 2 to 3 pounds for 2 or 3 days (See page 34.)

  - fatigue or tiredness that is much worse than you've had and that doesn't improve in 2 or 3 days

    - changes in heart rhythm that cause your heart to beat too fast or too slow or to skip around

      - severe bruising (for no known reason) or bleeding

Weight

Weigh yourself each day if you have had a problem with fluid retention since surgery or if you are on a low-salt diet or diuretic (water pill). A weight gain of 2 to 3 lbs. in one day is due to fluid, not fat. Call your doctor if you gain this amount of weight 2 days in a row.

- Weigh first thing in the morning after you urinate.
- Wear the same amount of clothes (or none) each time you weigh.
- Keep a daily record of your weight.

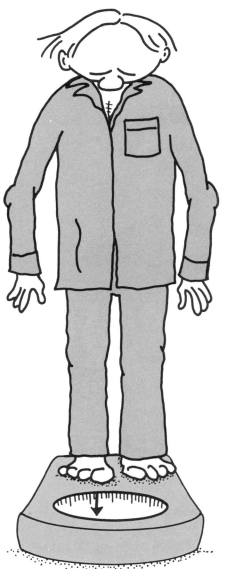

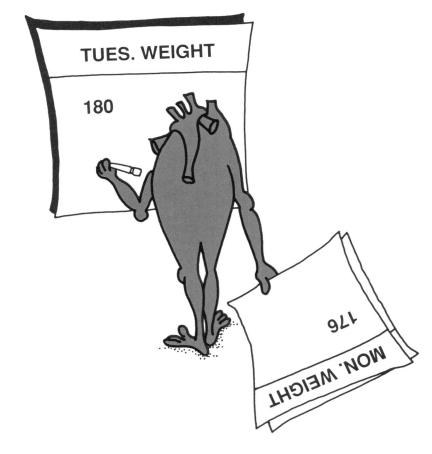

TUES. WEIGHT

180

176

MON. WEIGHT

Work

When you go back to work is most often decided after your 4 to 6 weeks checkup. It will depend on your **type of work,** the **demands** of your job, your level of **physical stamina** and other medical facts obtained from your checkup. It is not wise to make any major changes in your work plans or plan for your retirement until your recovery is complete.

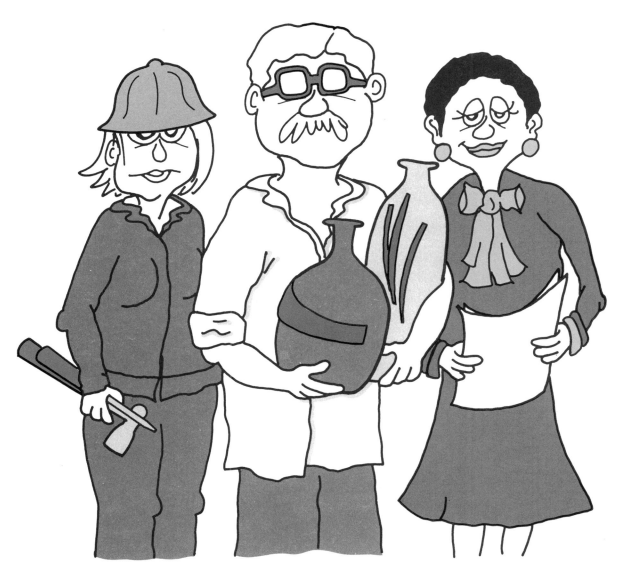

Each recovery is different.

More about your heart

Now that you know what to expect during recovery, this section will tell you more about your heart. It reviews normal heart function and the effect of diseases on the heart. It defines open heart surgery and reviews types of surgery that can improve heart function.

You will also learn what you can do to lower your chances of having more problems with your heart.

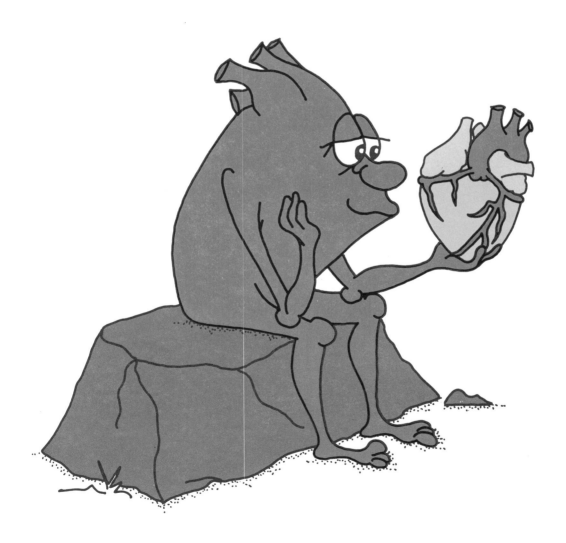

The heart and its chambers

The heart is a hollow, muscular organ about the size of a fist. It lies in the center of the chest, slightly to the left and is protected by the breastbone (sternum). The heart pumps blood, oxygen and nutrients to all parts of the body.

The heart is divided into 4 chambers. Two upper chambers (atria) receive blood from the veins. Two lower chambers (ventricles) pump blood out of the heart. Four valves in the heart act as one-way doors to direct blood flow. A wall (septum) divides the heart into a right and left side.

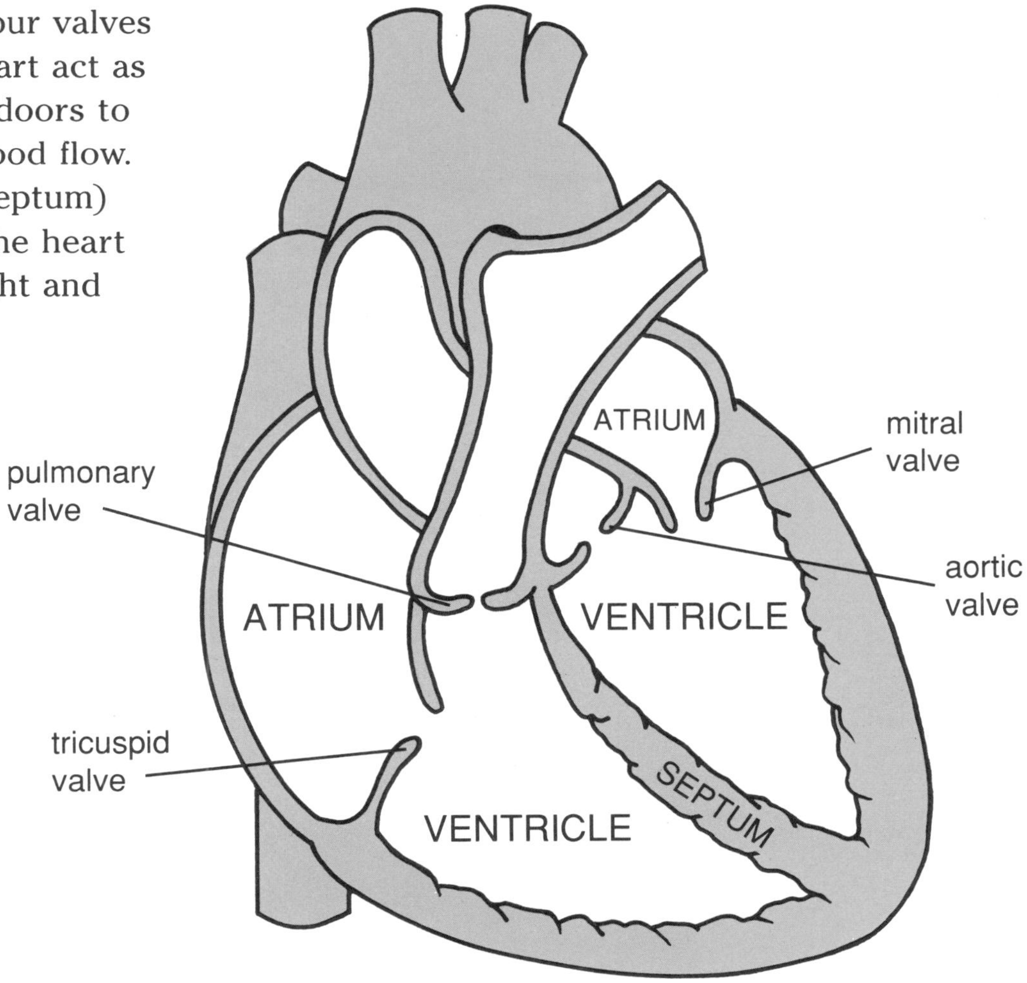

ATRIUM

mitral valve

pulmonary valve

aortic valve

ATRIUM

VENTRICLE

tricuspid valve

SEPTUM

VENTRICLE

The right and left sides of the heart

The right side of the heart receives blood from the body and pumps it to the lungs. This is the path the blood follows: body → veins → right atrium → tricuspid valve → right ventricle → pulmonary valve → pulmonary artery → lungs.

The left side of the heart receives oxygen-rich blood from the lungs and pumps it to the body. This is the path the blood follows: lungs → vein → left atrium → mitral valve → left ventricle → aortic valve → aorta → to all parts of the body.

This cycle is repeated about 70 times a minute and is counted as a pulse.

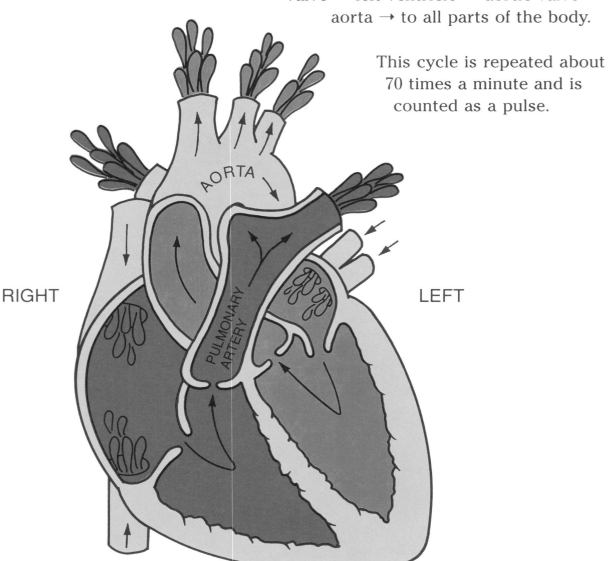

RIGHT

LEFT

Open heart surgery

Open heart surgery is done when normal heart function is changed by coronary artery disease, heart valve disease or other heart problems.

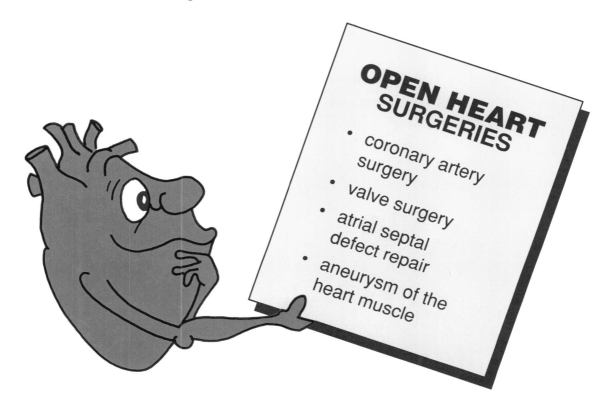

OPEN HEART SURGERIES
- coronary artery surgery
- valve surgery
- atrial septal defect repair
- aneurysm of the heart muscle

The term "open heart surgery" refers to any surgery in which the heart-lung or bypass machine is used. This machine pumps blood for the heart and adds oxygen for the lungs while the heart is at rest. Blood goes from the heart to the machine where it is cleaned, oxygenated and pumped back to the body. When the surgery is finished, the heart gradually takes over its job of pumping blood throughout the body.

The coronary arteries

The heart muscle is fed by the coronary arteries which start from the aorta. These arteries bring oxygen and nutrients to the heart muscle. Two main coronary arteries lie on the surface of the heart. They divide into smaller branches so that each part of the heart muscle receives nutrients.

The left coronary artery starts with a short part called the left main. It divides into the left anterior descending branch and the circumflex branch. The former feeds the left side and front of the heart muscle, and the circumflex takes blood to the back of the heart on the left side. The right coronary artery feeds the right side of the heart and has branches which extend to the back.

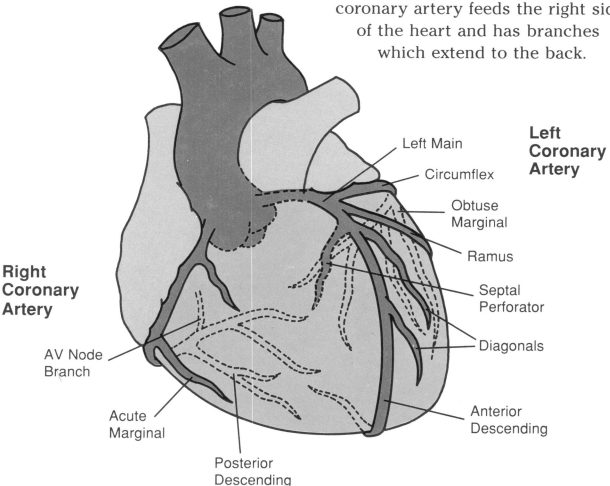

Left Coronary Artery

Left Main

Circumflex

Obtuse Marginal

Ramus

Septal Perforator

Diagonals

Anterior Descending

Right Coronary Artery

AV Node Branch

Acute Marginal

Posterior Descending

Coronary artery disease

The coronary arteries can become narrowed by a buildup of fatty layers in the artery walls (atherosclerosis)*. As a result, less blood flows through the arteries. If 75% of a coronary artery is blocked, the heart muscle may not get enough blood and oxygen. When this happens, angina may occur.

Angina

Angina warns that the heart is not getting enough blood and oxygen. Symptoms include: *pressure, tightness, squeezing, aching, burning* or *cramping* in the chest, arm, neck or jaw or *shortness of breath*. You can have angina when the heart is working harder than usual during exercise, when excited and after eating. You can also have angina when resting.

The quickest way to relieve angina is with nitroglycerin (NTG) and rest. Damage to the heart muscle (a heart attack) can occur if angina is not relieved and lasts more than 15 minutes. Symptoms of a heart attack are like angina but often more intense.

* Atherosclerosis is one type of arteriosclerosis, the medical term for "hardening of the arteries."

Coronary artery surgery

Coronary artery surgery is done to bypass one or more blockages in the coronary arteries. The bypass increases blood flow to the heart muscle to relieve angina and improve heart function. A leg vein (saphenous vein) or an artery from the chest (internal mammary artery) can be used for the bypass graft. The type of graft used depends on the number and location of your blockages.

When a leg vein is used, one end is sewn to the aorta and the other end to the coronary artery below the blockage. Using a leg vein does not bother blood flow to that area of your leg or your ability to walk.

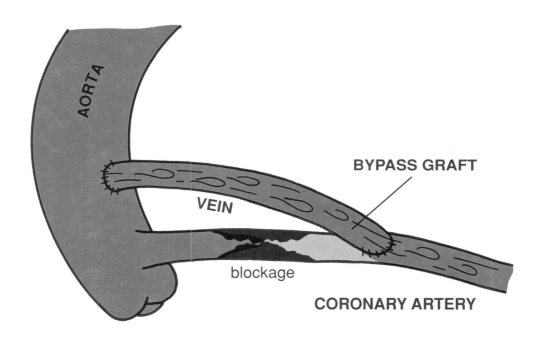

When an internal mammary artery is used (p. 43, Fig. 1), one end is left attached to a branch of the aorta. The other end is sewn to the coronary artery below the blockage. Oxygen-rich blood flows through the graft to the heart muscle.

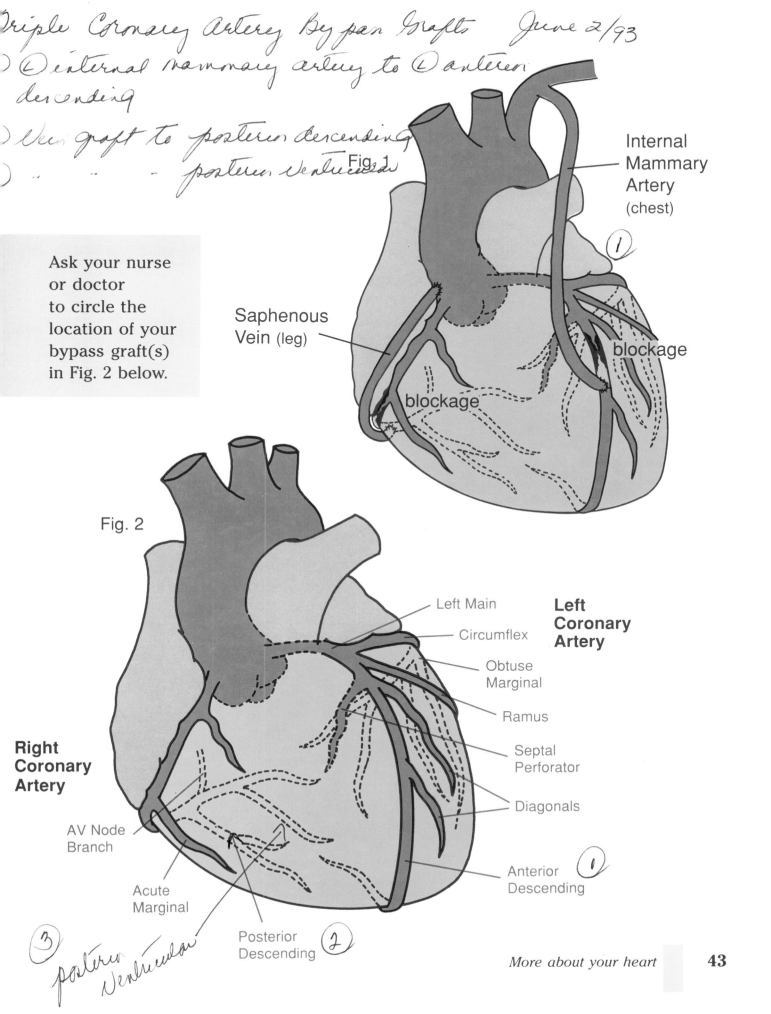

Triple Coronary Artery Bypass Grafts   June 2/93
1) internal mammary artery to 1) anterior descending
2) Vein graft to posterior descending
3) .... - posterior ventricular

Fig. 1

Internal
Mammary
Artery
(chest)

Saphenous
Vein (leg)

blockage

blockage

Ask your nurse
or doctor
to circle the
location of your
bypass graft(s)
in Fig. 2 below.

Fig. 2

Left Main

Circumflex

**Left
Coronary
Artery**

Obtuse
Marginal

Ramus

Septal
Perforator

Diagonals

Anterior
Descending

**Right
Coronary
Artery**

AV Node
Branch

Acute
Marginal

Posterior
Descending

posterior
ventricular

Risk factors

Certain risks are known to increase your chances of having artery blockages in the future. The 3 major risk factors for coronary artery disease are:

- **smoking**
- eating a lot of **saturated fat**
- **high blood pressure**

Other risks that raise the oxygen and pumping demands on the heart are:

- **obesity** (more than 20% overweight)
- tension or **stress**
- **lack of exercise**

Also, people with **diabetes** or a **family history** of heart disease are at greater risk for heart disease.

SMOKE	EAT HIGH-FAT	OVER WEIGHT	HIGH BP	LITTLE/NO EXERCISE
DON'T SMOKE	EAT LOW-FAT	GOOD BODY WEIGHT	CONTROLLED BP	EXERCISE 3-4 TIMES A WEEK

YOU make the choices.

See page 51.

Heart valve disease

Normal heart valves are thin, smooth structures that direct blood through the heart's chambers. The valves can be changed or damaged by birth defects, infection, rheumatic fever or scarlet fever. Over time, scarring or thickening can occur. With these changes, the valves are harder to open (stenosis) or can't close all the way (insufficiency). The aortic and mitral valves are the ones most often damaged. These valves control blood flow through the main pumping chamber.

When valves do not open and close as they should, less blood gets through. This causes the heart to work harder to pump blood to the body. If the heart is not able to do this, heart failure occurs. Abnormal valves can also cause an irregular heartbeat or blood clots to form in the heart.

With heart failure, blood is not emptied out of the heart. It backs up into the lungs and other body parts. As a result, shortness of breath, swelling, coughing or extreme tiredness occur.

At times, medications improve the heart's pumping and relieve the heart failure. But surgery is often needed to improve the heart's function.

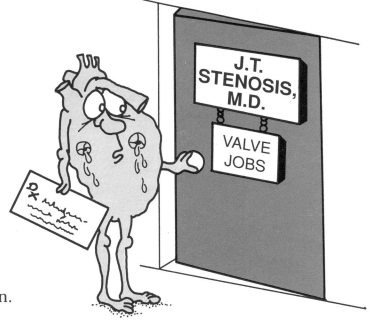

Heart valve surgery

When possible, your own heart valve is repaired. More often, the damaged heart valve must be replaced. Some people feel better right after surgery since their symptoms are relieved. But for most people it is a few months before they feel the benefits of heart valve surgery. It takes time for the heart to recover from the extra work it was doing before surgery. For this reason, your doctor may ask you to keep taking medicines and to follow a special diet.

If the valve is replaced, it will be with either a mechanical or tissue valve. The tissue valve may be porcine (heterograft) or human (homograft). Here are just a few of the valves that can be used. Yours may be a little different from the ones shown here.

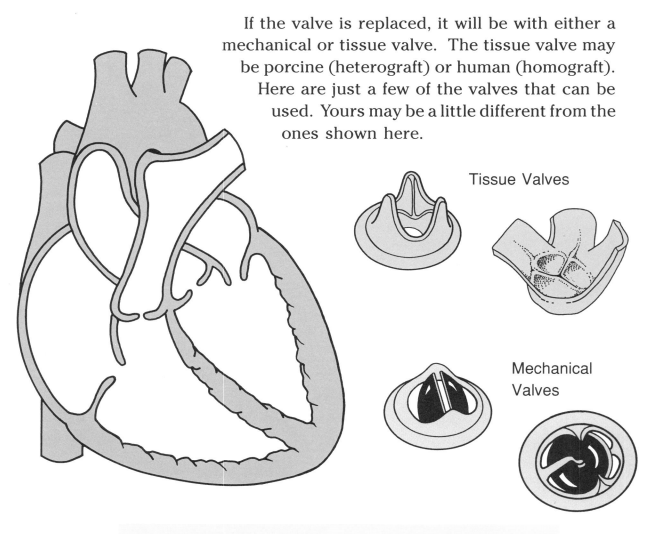

Tissue Valves

Mechanical Valves

Ask your nurse or doctor to write in the name of the valve used (_____) and circle its location.

Prevention of bacterial endocarditis

Bacterial endocarditis is very serious. It is an infection of the valves and/or inner heart lining (endocardium). It can damage or destroy heart valves.

Bacterial endocarditis can occur when bacteria enter the bloodstream during infections, dental work, surgery, procedures or IV injections with dirty needles. Anyone who has a **heart defect, heart valve disease** or has had **heart valve surgery is at high risk** for this infection.

CAUTION

Taking antibiotics may reduce your risk of infection. Ask your doctor to prescribe antibiotics before having any of these:

- **ALL dental work:** routine cleaning, filling or removing teeth, gum work, root canals or treatment of mouth ulcers

- **any major surgery**

- **minor surgeries** such as: drainage of an abscess, tonsillectomy, appendectomy, prostate surgery and, in some cases, childbirth

- **procedures which cause trauma to body tissues:** bladder exams, some rectal and colon exams

Symptoms of endocarditis can be vague. Call your doctor if you have fever, sweating, chills, loss of appetite or tiredness that does not go away in 2 to 3 days. Bacterial endocarditis is treated with antibiotics. Blood samples should be drawn for culture before any antibiotics are given.

Anticoagulants

Some people get blood clots inside an artery, a vein or the heart. This may be a problem in people with mechanical heart valves, irregular heartbeats or previous blood clots. To lower the chance of having blood clots, an anticoagulant (such as Coumadin) is prescribed.

Anticoagulants (commonly called "blood thinners") lengthen the time it normally takes for blood to clot. If you are taking a blood thinner, **keep appointments for a regular blood test** (prothrombin time). The "pro time" tells your doctor how long it takes your blood to clot. This time is used to decide the right dose of blood thinner for you. While you are in the hospital, your blood will most likely be checked daily. When you first go home, a prothrombin time should be done once a week. Later, this may be needed only once a month.

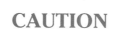 **CAUTION** Watch for signs of bleeding if you are taking a blood thinner. Let your doctor know right away if you see:

- black bowel movements
- pink or red urine
- excessive bruising or unexplained swelling
- severe headaches or abdominal pain
- vomitus that looks like coffee grounds
- heavy nose bleeds
- heavy menstrual periods

Do not use aspirin or any medicine that contains aspirin (Bufferin, Excedrin, Alka-Seltzer, cold remedies, etc.) while taking a blood thinner. This could lead to bleeding. Read all labels.

Acetaminophen (Tylenol, Datril, Anacin-3, etc.) prescribed by your doctor may be used for minor aches, pains and headaches.

Take only the drugs prescribed by your doctor. Many over-the-counter drugs can change how your blood thinner works.

If dental work or surgery is planned, let the dentist or surgeon know you are on anticoagulants. Your doctor may ask you to stop taking them for a time.

If taking a long trip, tell your doctor so plans for blood tests can be made while you are away.

Carry ID (identification) showing that you are taking anticoagulants.

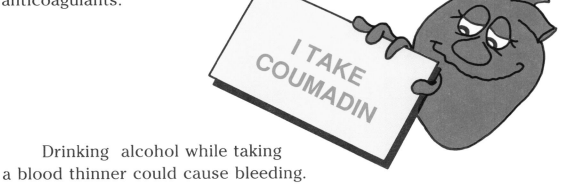

Drinking alcohol while taking a blood thinner could cause bleeding. Check with your doctor about using alcohol.

Do not play contact sports (football, soccer, rugby, etc.). Injuries often occur with these sports that would cause bleeding.

Take your blood thinner exactly as prescribed by your doctor. **NEVER** stop taking your blood thinner on your own.

You may also have heart surgery for an atrial septal defect or aneurysm of the heart muscle.

Atrial septal defect

Sometimes at birth, the wall that divides the heart's upper chambers does not close all the way. This leaves a hole that lets blood flow between the upper chambers. Problems with respiratory infections, fatigue, shortness of breath or irregular heartbeats can occur. In surgery, the hole is either sewn together or patched with pericardium or a synthetic material.

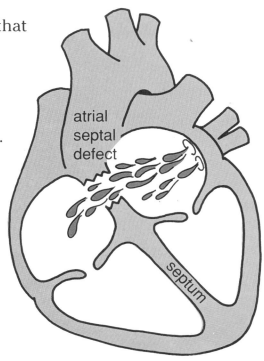

Aneurysm of the heart muscle

Bulging of the heart muscle (ventricular aneurysm) can happen after a heart attack. If this happens, the heart does not pump as well. You may have shortness of breath, pain or irregular heartbeats. In surgery, the bulge is cut out or patched.

Notes & Resources

Risk factors

List the risk factors in your life and your goals for reducing them. Check your answers by page 44.

Risk factor

Goals

Walk exercise

	1st week at home	2nd week at home	3rd week at home
Time			
Times/Day			
Pace			

Walk at an easy pace. It may make you a little winded, but do not let it make you too short of breath to talk (the "talk test"). If you take your pulse, it should not increase more than _____. If your pulse increases more than this, slow down.

Talk to your doctor about your progress and adjust your walks as he or she suggests.

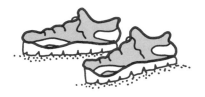

Stationary bike exercise

	1st week at home	2nd week at home	3rd week at home
Time			
Frequency			
Tension			
Speed			

Talk about your progress with your doctor or cardiac rehab team.

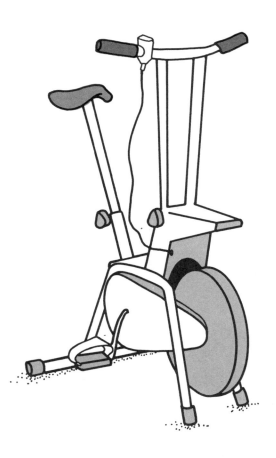

Medications

List the medicines you will take at home.
(Your nurse or doctor can help you fill this in.)

name	how much/how often	times			

Review pages 22-23 about medicines. Review pages 48-49 if you are taking an anticoagulant.

Know what any drug you take does and the possible side effects it could have.

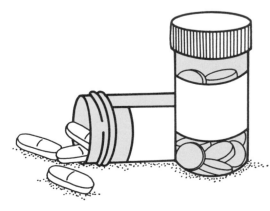

Checklist *(for you or your family)*

It's hard to remember all you are told in the hospital. Make notes here before you go home, and get answers to your questions.

List the things that you normally do but should not do until your doctor says it is OK. (See pp. 20-21.)

_____   _____
_____   _____
_____   _____
_____   _____
_____   _____

Look at p. 24. Some of the activities that you like or want to do may not be listed on this page. Write those here, and ask your doctor or nurse if and when these will be OK for you.

_____   _____
_____   _____
_____   _____
_____   _____
_____   _____

My next appointment is:

_____
_____

Doctor: **Phone Number:**

_____   _____
_____   _____
_____   _____

Know what symptoms to watch for and when to call your doctor. (Review pp. 32-33.)

Other books to help your heart

It's Heartly Fare © 1991
A food book that makes sense of fat, cholesterol and salt
Order from:
Pritchett & Hull Associates, Inc.
(not available in bookstores)

American Heart Association
Low-Fat, Low-Cholesterol Cookbook © 1989
Order from:
Pritchett & Hull
(also available in major bookstores)

Don't Eat Your Heart Out Cookbook © 1982
Choices For A Healthy Heart © 1987
by Joseph C. Piscatella
Order from:
Pritchett & Hull
(also available in major bookstores)

Light & Healthy Microwave Cooking © 1986
by J. Emal & E. Taylor, R.D.
Order from:
Pritchett & Hull
(also available in major bookstores)

Exercise for Heart & Health © 1985
Order from:
Pritchett & Hull
(not available in bookstores)

The Relaxation Response © 1975
by Herbert Benson, M.D.
(available in major bookstores)

Blood Pressure Control © 1988
Order from:
Pritchett & Hull Associates, Inc.
(not available in bookstores)

These are only a few of the books available to help you toward a more healthy heart and lifestyle. There are also many tapes and videos on weight control, stopping smoking, exercise, etc. Look in your local bookstore and video store for subjects that would be helpful for you. Your doctor or nurse may also have some suggestions.